PRESENTED TO

MARES MEMORIAL LIBRARY

BY

CITIZENS STATE BANK

IN MEMORY OF

MRS. FRANK TODORA

BEYOND 2000
THE HEALTH REVOLUTION

Surgery and Medicine in the Twenty-first Century

BEYOND 2000

THE HEALTH REVOLUTION

Surgery and Medicine in the Twenty-first Century

by David Darling

Dillon Press
Parsippany, New Jersey

Acknowledgments

The author wishes to thank Seymour Schwartz, M.D., Professor and Chair, Department of Surgery, University of Rochester, for his expert comments during the preparation of this book.

Photo Credits

COVER: © James Stevenson/Science Photo Library/Photo Researchers, Inc.

© CNRI/Science Photo Library/Photo Researchers, Inc.: 17. © Department of Clinical Radiology, Salisbury District Hospital/Science Photo Library/Photo Researchers, Inc.: 10, 42. © Simon Fraser/Science Photo Library/Photo Researchers, Inc.: 11. © Simon Fraser/Department of Neuroradiology, Newcastle General Hospital/Science Photo Library/Photo Researchers, Inc.: 13. © Stevie Grand/Science Photo Library/Photo Researchers, Inc.: 31. © David Guyon, The BOC Group PLC/Science Photo Library/Photo Researchers, Inc.: 32. © Philippe Plailly/Science Photo Library/Photo Researchers, Inc.: 15. © Chris Priest/Science Photo Library/Photo Researchers, Inc.: 35. © Princess Margaret Rose Orthopaedic Hospital/Science Photo Library/Photo Researchers, Inc.: 45. © St. Bartholomew's Hospital/Science Photo Library/Photo Researchers, Inc.: 48. © Science Photo Library/Photo Researchers, Inc.: 43. © Jim Stevenson/Science Photo Library/Photo Researchers, Inc.: 25. © Geoff Tompkinson/Science Photo Library/Photo Researchers, Inc.: 20, 26. David A. Wagner/Phototake NYC: 5. Illustrations by Christine Schaar: 22, 27, 36, 52, 54.

Library of Congress Cataloging-in-Publication Data

Darling, David J.
The health revolution : surgery and medicine in the twenty-first century / by David Darling. — 1st ed.
p. cm. — (Beyond 2000)
Includes bibliographical references and index.
ISBN 0-87518-616-5 (lsb). — ISBN 0-382-39170-5 (pbk.)
1. Surgery—Technological innovations—Juvenile literature. 2. Artificial organs—Juvenile literature. 3. Prosthesis—Juvenile literature. 4. Medical innovations—Juvenile literature.
[1. Medical innovations. 2. Artificial organs. 3. Prosthesis.]
I. Title. II. Series.
RD31.5.D37 1996
610'.28—dc20 95-14223

Summary: Describes current and possible future advances in surgical techniques and the development of medical devices and artificial body parts.

Published by Dillon Press,
A Division of Simon & Schuster,
299 Jefferson Road, Parisppany, NJ 07054

First edition

Printed in the United States of America

10 9 8 7 6 5 4 3 2 1

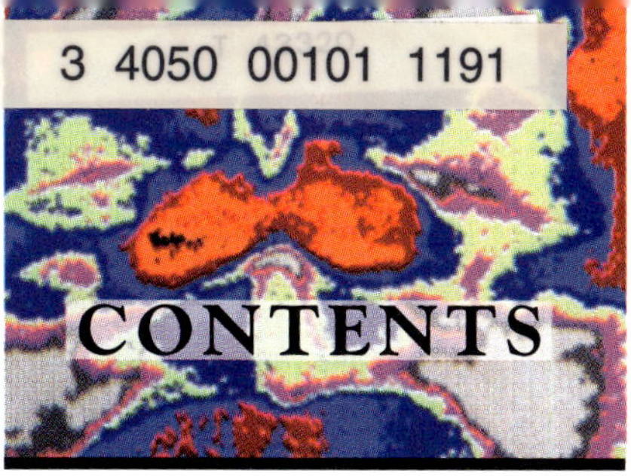

CONTENTS

Introduction

In times past the more blood a surgeon got on his gown, the more highly he was regarded. Since there were no anesthetics to numb patients or make them unconscious, even simple operations were incredibly painful. Surgeons worked as fast as they could in an effort to prevent their patients from simply dying of shock. Often, the surgeons took gruesome pride in being able to saw off diseased limbs in a matter of seconds. This earned them the common nickname "sawbones." A range of primitive-looking tools that would have seemed more at home in a butcher's hands were all that the surgeon had to work with, and cleanliness was considered unimportant. Many patients who survived their operations died shortly afterward because their wounds became infected.

Thankfully, the days of the sawbones are long gone. Patients today are given effective anesthetics, and operating rooms are kept scrupulously clean. Surgical personnel wear sterilized gowns, masks, and boots, and go through a meticulous "scrubbing up" procedure before donning sterile surgical gloves. All instruments are made germ-free by being placed in an autoclave, a small oven that bathes them in super-hot steam.

But until recently many of the tools of the early surgeons—with minor improvements—were still used for most operations. Only within the last 15 years or so has surgery begun to be transformed by high-technology devices. Among these are precision lasers for making bloodless cuts, special flexible probes and tools that can be passed through button-sized holes into the patient's body, and instruments for doing operations on a microscopic scale.

Other breakthroughs have been made in the field of spare-part surgery. Every year, doctors replace an increasing number of body parts with artificial substitutes. The techniques for carrying out organ transplants are also being improved and extended.

Great strides have been made in the methods and machinery designed to save people's lives. And some particularly exciting developments have taken place in the technology of scanning equipment used to look closely at internal parts of the human body for early signs of diseases such as cancer.

Not surprisingly, given these advances, surgeons today can successfully operate to cure all sorts of complaints that not so long ago would have been difficult or impossible to treat. Many more advancements in surgery will take place in the years ahead as new instruments, materials, and techniques are developed. The revolution in the hospital and the operating room has just begun.

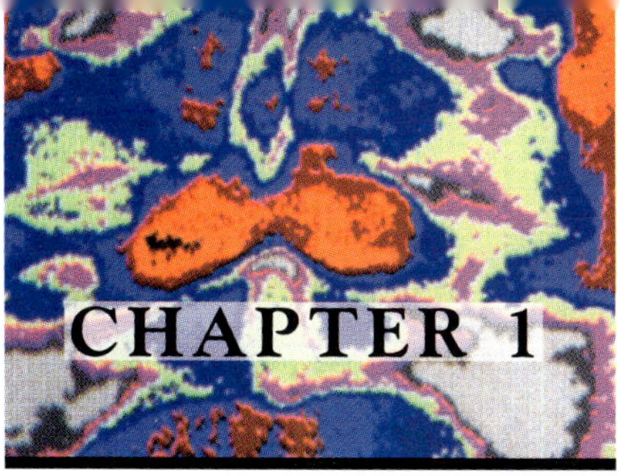

CHAPTER 1

Looking for Trouble

Fifty years ago the main way to see inside a person's body without cutting it open involved taking an X-ray photograph. **X-rays*** were discovered in 1895 by a German-born Dutch citizen, William Roentgen. X-rays pass fairly easily through the soft parts of the human body but are stopped by harder or more dense parts. So when a beam of X-rays is passed through a person's body and onto a photographic plate, solid objects such as bone show up in white on a negative print. This makes X-ray photos ideal for seeing details of fractures and dislocations without opening the body.

However, bones are not the only body parts that X-rays can reveal. For example, if a special dyelike chemical is first introduced into soft **tissues***, such as an artery, the intestine, or the

Words that appear in* ***bold* *are explained in the glossary on page 57.*

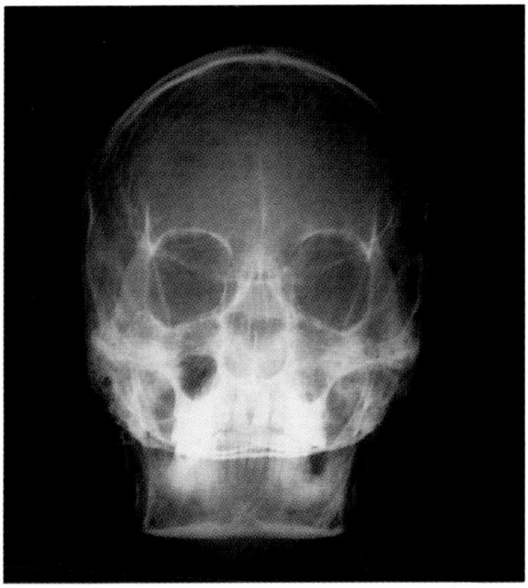

An X-ray photograph of a human skull

stomach, the chemical absorbs the X-rays and shows more clearly the shapes and positions of the soft structures. In this way, major blood vessels and **organs** can be observed to check for signs of damage or disease. Ordinary X-ray methods, however, are very limited in what they can show.

CAT's Eye View

In 1967 a British engineer, Geoffrey Hounslow, realized that computers were the key to providing a much better view of the inside of the human body. He devised a system called **CAT** (computerized axial tomography). This system works by directing a series of narrow X-ray beams through the patient to produce detailed cross sections. A computer then combines the cross sections to build up a three-dimensional picture—a CAT scan—in which different tissues are distinguished by how well they block X-rays or let them through. The computer uses a range of colors to show up tissues and organs according to their density. Then it displays the processed image on a video monitor.

The earliest CAT scanners were fixed in position and took 30 seconds or so to produce the image of a single cross section. But as computers became more and more powerful, the performance

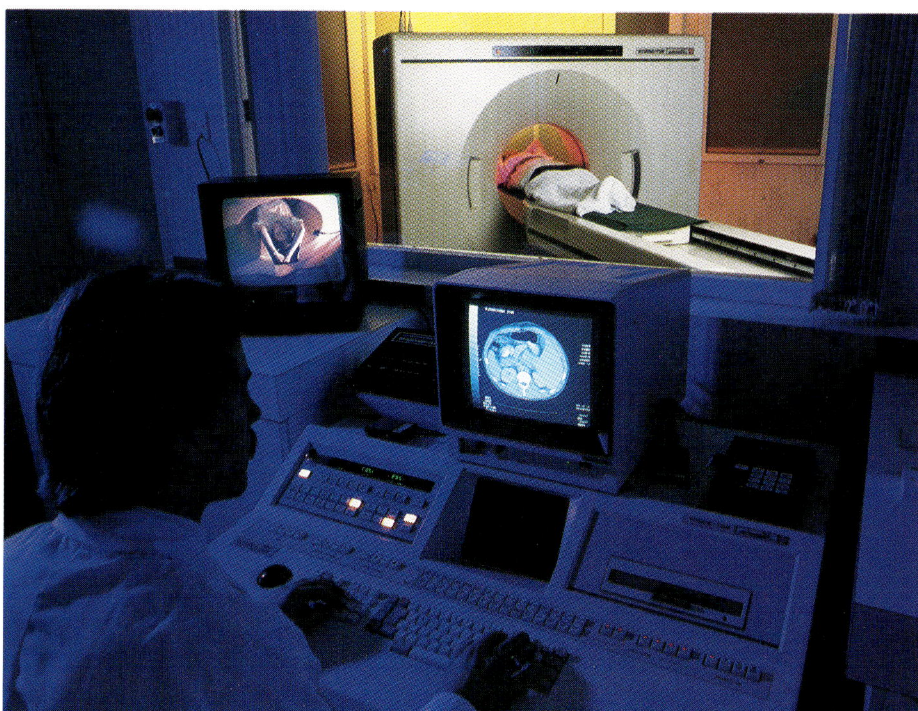

A CAT scan in progress, showing the scanner and patient in the background and the radiographer working at the scanner's computer terminal in the foreground. An image of the patient's abdomen appears on the screen.

of CAT scanners improved dramatically. The latest devices, which use rotating machinery and scan in a spiral pattern, can produce an image slice every second. Such sophisticated, high-speed scanning allows doctors to track the passage of injected substances through blood vessels and into organs and **tumors**.

The main drawback of a CAT scanner is its use of X-rays, which in large doses can be harmful to the patient. This is particularly true if the patient is a child. For this reason, although CAT scanners are still widely used at present and will remain important for studying organs such as the lungs, stomach, and intestines, they are likely to give way to other scanning methods in the future.

Scanning Without X-rays

The basic idea of the CAT scanner, to build three-dimensional pictures from many cross sections with the help of a computer, is now used in several other types of scanners. The **PET** (positron emission tomography) scanner, for instance, is used to identify and monitor problems with the brain. Patients are injected with a solution of glucose (a type of sugar) and a tiny amount of **radioactive** material. As the glucose reaches the brain, different areas of the brain take up varying amounts of the sugar, depending on the energy needs of those areas. How much energy a part of the brain needs depends on its level of activity. The PET scanner detects the radiation coming from the radioactive glucose and so allows a picture of brain activity to be built up. This enables doctors to look for the distinctive patterns of activity associated with specific brain disorders, such as **Alzheimer's disease**.

An even more advanced method of producing pictures of what is going on inside the body is **MRI** (magnetic resonance imaging). This technique is based on the fact that **hydrogen atoms** in the body give off radio waves at a special **frequency** after having been bombarded with other, high-frequency radio waves and subjected to a powerful **magnetic field**.

As does a CAT scanner, the MRI machine enables doctors to view three-dimensional images of the body on a screen. But MRI can be used when X-rays might be considered too hazardous to the patient. It is especially useful for monitoring the progress of diseases such as muscular dystrophy (a muscle-wasting condition) and of patients who have undergone operations involving organ **transplants**.

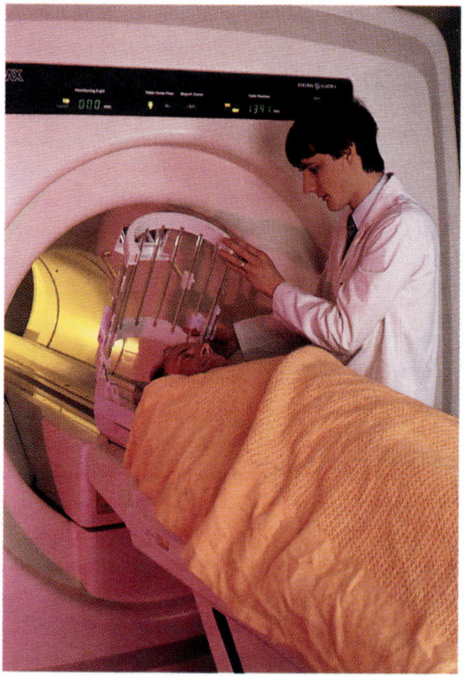

A patient being prepared for an MRI scan. The patient's head is surrounded by the coils of the scanner's magnet; the smaller device above the patient's head is a radio frequency receiver.

Recently, MRI has been applied to the study of muscle injuries. Even when injured muscles are no longer painful, MRI images show tissue repair continuing for up to three weeks. This suggests that before resuming heavy training and competition, athletes with muscle injuries should take a longer period to recover than previously believed necessary.

A great deal of research and development is going on to improve MRI technology, and it is likely that this method of scanning will become increasingly important in the future. MRI scanners will become less expensive, and as a result more hospitals will be able to afford them. At the same time, the equipment will become smaller and capable of producing higher-quality images. This will lead to the technique's being applied in new ways, such as the imaging of blood vessels and of very small tumors.

Medicine by Numbers

Today, doctors are making more and more use of **digital images**—pictures built up from numbers that have been processed by a computer. Digital X-rays and pictures produced by various types of scanning machines may eventually make conventional X-ray film obsolete.

Much more can be done with picture information stored in a computer than with simple X-ray photographs. A doctor can create a three-dimensional model of a patient's organs, soft tissues, or bones and then rotate or slice through this model in

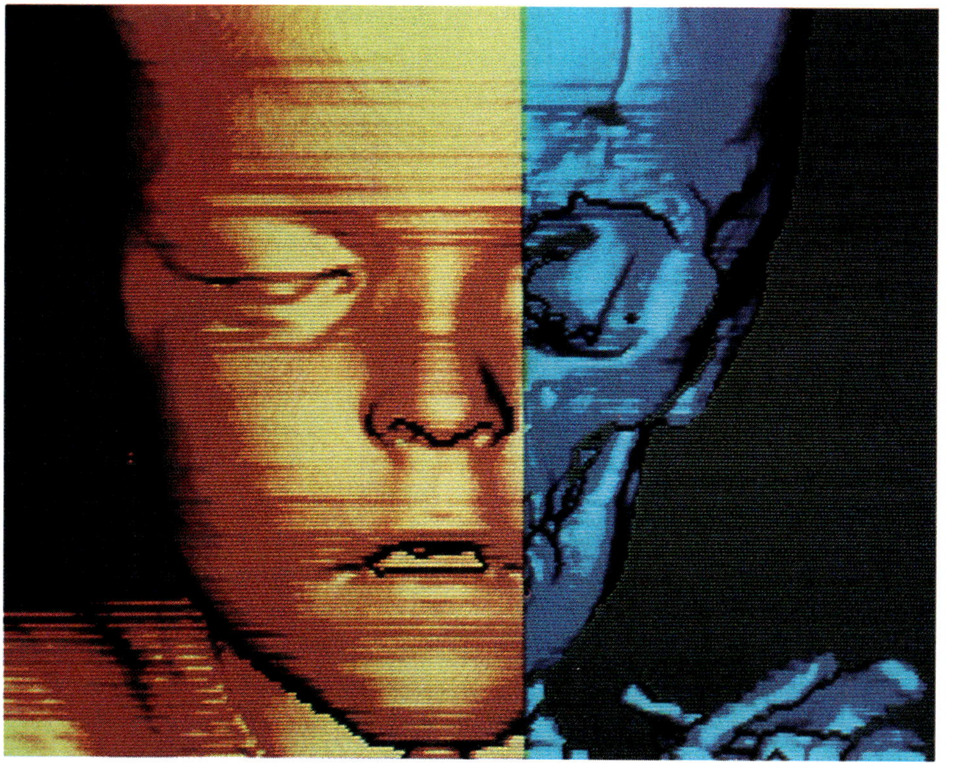

A three-dimensional reconstruction of a child's face obtained from CAT scan data, showing the skin surface on the left and the underlying skull on the right

various ways at a computer workstation. Output from the computer can be used to manufacture accurately shaped artificial body parts. Using the computer, surgeons can practice a new or difficult type of operation before carrying out the procedure on a patient. Medical students can study the layout of the body and the appearance of various diseases in a totally new way.

Another great benefit of digital images over conventional X-rays is that digital images can be produced using a much lower dose of radiation. This reduces the chance of any harmful side effects to the patient. Also, information in digital form can be sent easily from one computer to another. For example, detailed pictures of a patient in one location can be studied by a surgeon at a computer workstation in another city or country.

In the future, images produced by a variety of different devices, such as CAT and MRI scanners, will be combined to reveal even more details of the body's internal structure. This process will be extended to control the delivery of treatment. At a computer workstation, doctors will merge all the image information about a patient's condition with the most appropriate surgical procedure, including details of the instruments and techniques to be used. The computer will then generate all the information needed to direct needles, lasers, and even robotic surgical tools under the remote guidance of the surgeon.

Sound Probe

An unborn baby, or **fetus**, in its mother's womb resembles a submerged submarine—a similarity that triggered an idea by a Scottish medical professor, Ian Donald, in the 1950s. To study the fetus, Donald and his colleagues borrowed a technique called sonar, developed by French, British, and American scientists during World War II to detect enemy vessels and other objects underwater. The medical professors realized that, when adapted, sonar could be used to check the progress of a fetus during pregnancy.

Sonar is based on the fact that very high pitched sound waves, known as **ultrasound**, travel particularly well through water and similar liquids and send back clear echoes from any solid object they meet. The echoes can be converted into a picture of the object and displayed on a screen.

Great advances have been made in ultrasound methods over the past 40 years, to the extent that roughly a quarter of all medical imaging carried out in hospitals now involves this technique. Because experience has shown that ultrasound is less harmful than X-rays and other types of radiation, it is used routinely to check on the health of fetuses. But it is also applied in many other ways. Ultrasound devices have been made in hundreds of specialized forms. Some scan organs from outside the body, and others are inserted through holes in the body to scan blood vessels and organs such as the heart, the stomach, and the intestines.

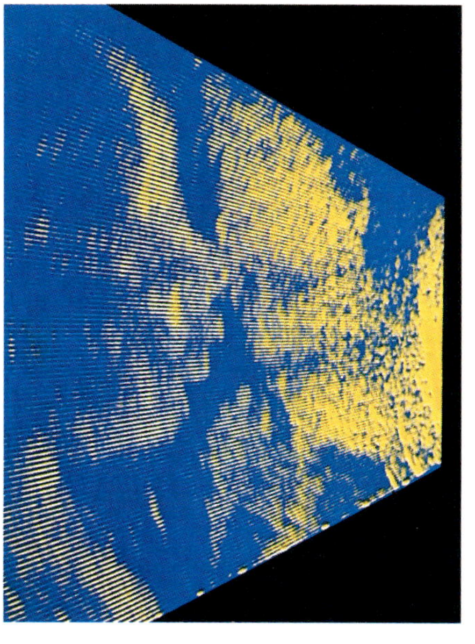

An ultrasound picture of a seven-month-old fetus in its mother's womb, showing the face and shoulders in profile

An adaptation of the ultrasound method, called **Doppler scanning**, can be used to measure how fast blood is flowing through a patient's arteries and veins and so can help to detect any blockages in blood vessels.

With further progress in the miniaturization of equipment, the ultrasound technique will be applied in even more varied ways. As the scanning method of first choice when infants and young children are involved, it will be used increasingly in procedures such as heart and brain surgery in newborn babies. It will also be employed more and more frequently to monitor in adults those parts of the body, for example, the prostate gland, that are particularly sensitive to exposure to X-rays and other radiation.

Murmuring Muscles

The fact that muscles make low-frequency sounds when they contract has been known for over three centuries, but until recently nothing useful had come of this knowledge. Within the past few years, however, researchers have begun to exploit the medical potential of muscle sounds. When an electronic stethoscope is attached to a body area such as the arm, the sound produced by contracting muscles is fed to an amplifier and a special computer. This computer separates the various components of the sounds and produces a visible record of its findings. Doctors can then study the results to look for telltale sounds made by torn or strained muscles. The same technique may eventually be used to detect abnormalities of the heart—the most important muscle-containing structure in the body.

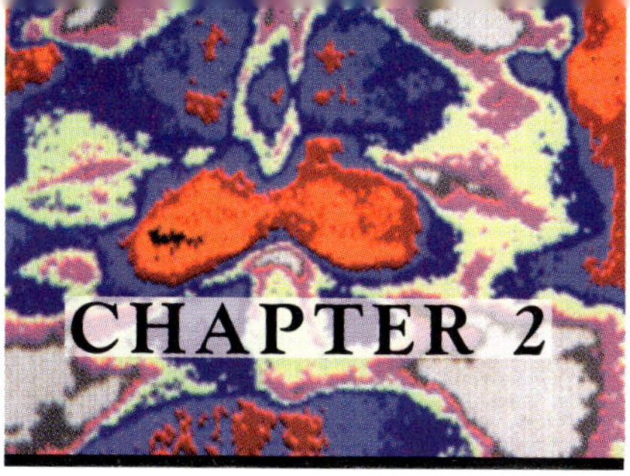

CHAPTER 2

Operating on a Small Scale

Until quite recently most operations followed a similar pattern. The surgeon would make a generous incision through a patient's skin with a sharp instrument called a **scalpel** and then hold the cut open with separating tools called **retractors**. Next the surgeon would pinch off severed blood vessels with **forceps**, and, if necessary, saw through bone to reach the problem area. Some operations must still be carried out in this way. But now the emphasis in surgery has shifted to doing as little damage to the patient as possible. This type of surgery is known as **minimum-intervention** surgery and, among other techniques, involves passing instruments into the body through very small incisions and using new devices such as surgical lasers to avoid making unnecessary cuts.

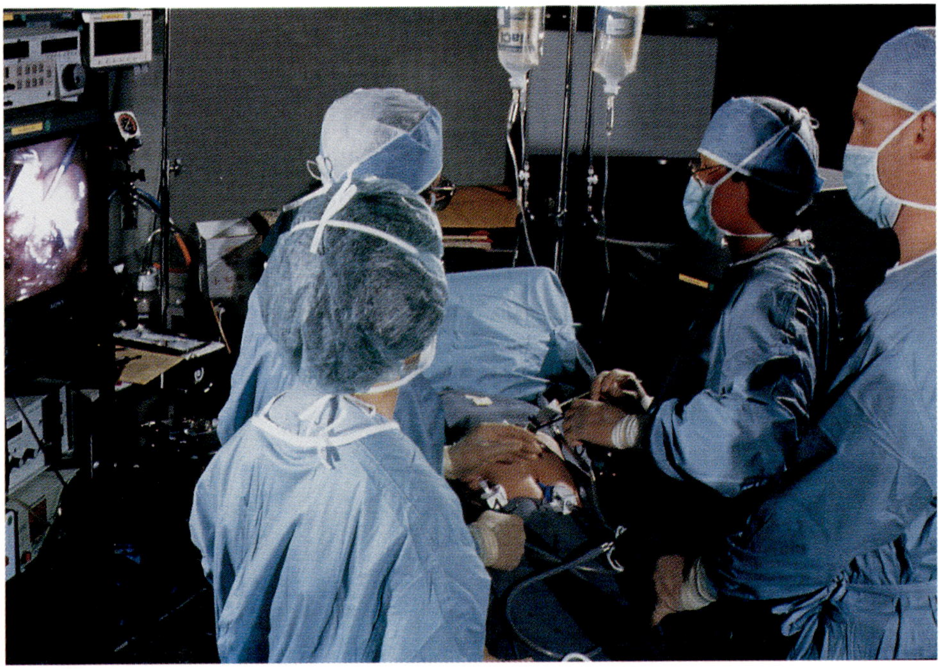

Surgeons remove a patient's gallbladder through a tiny incision, using a laser beam and other minimal-intervention techniques. The operation is viewed on a TV monitor.

A View Through the Keyhole

Operating through cuts that may be only an inch or so across has given rise to the name **keyhole surgery**. An instrument called an **endoscope** enables surgeons to see what they are doing through such narrow openings.

The first endoscope, said to have been invented by Phillipe Bozzini of Frankfurt, Germany, in 1806, was just a narrow, rigid tube down which a light could be shone. With it, a doctor would have been able, for instance, to get a rather murky view of the inside of a patient's throat or stomach.

But endoscopes have been improved a great deal since those early days. Now they are made from **optical fibers**—fine, flexible strands of special glass or plastic along which light can travel for long distances and even around bends. Light is shone down one bundle of optical fibers, and the surgeon sees through another bundle, which is equipped with a strong lens. Also running down the length of the endoscope are control wires that allow the surgeon to guide and maneuver the instrument from outside the patient's body. Light traveling along the fiber-optic bundles relays a picture to a viewing device held in front of the surgeon or onto a video screen, enabling the surgeon and others to watch what is happening.

Surgery in a Tight Spot

In addition to giving an amazingly clear view of the inside of the body, an endoscope can also carry instruments to perform certain types of operations. Because of the limited space within the endoscope's tube, however, none of these instruments can be more than about 3 millimeters in diameter, and all must be long and flexible. Examples include tiny cutting devices and forceps to cut away, grip, and pull away unwanted tissue (some of which may be analyzed in the laboratory); minute **electrodes** through which an electric current can be passed to seal blood vessels; and small balloons that can be used to open stuck heart valves.

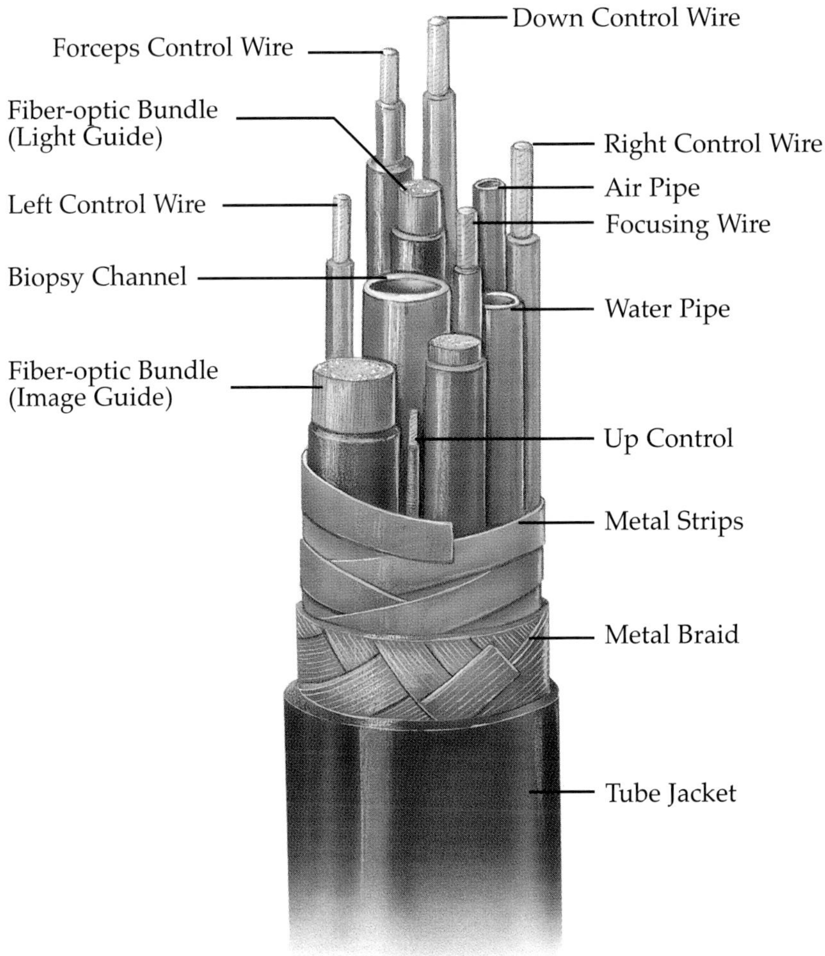

Endoscopes help surgeons to see inside the body and perform surgery through very small incisions by remote control. With fine, flexible tubes, the surgeon can see around bends. Light travels down one bundle of optical fibers, and the surgeon views through another bundle. Wires control the instrument from outside the body. Pipes carry air and water.

Laser beams can also be directed down optical fibers in an endoscope to control bleeding, make bloodless cuts through tissue (since the heat from the laser immediately seals the wound), and destroy tumors and other growths inside the body.

Smaller even than the openings made during keyhole surgery are those used in another new technique, called **percutaneous surgery**. *Percutaneous* simply means "through the skin." It involves making a tiny hole through the patient's skin and muscle with a needle just 1 millimeter across. Using a series of wider tubes, the surgeon temporarily stretches the hole until it is a few millimeters across. During this procedure, instead of muscles and other tissues of the body being cut, they are just gently forced apart. Since hardly any blood is lost by the patient, no **blood transfusions** are needed, and no wounds that require stitches are left behind. The patient recovers almost immediately and may be able to leave the hospital less than a day after the operation.

Unlike the flexible tools used with ordinary endoscopes, percutaneous instruments are rigid. They are often merely modified or scaled-down versions of standard surgical instruments. Many were originally designed for operating on the ear.

Microsurgery

Today if a person's arm, leg, fingers, or toes are accidentally cut off, they can sometimes be reattached and made to work again, thanks to advances in surgery. Simply reattaching

Small-scale Surgery on the Spine

Slipped disks in the back are now routinely treated by percutaneous surgery. A disk is a doughnut-shaped piece of cartilage (a tough, gristly substance) that fits between the bones in a person's spine and acts like the suspension system of a car. Fluid surrounding each disk also serves to absorb shock waves that travel up the spine when a person moves around. Disks do not actually "slip." The cartilage simply gets worn and, as a result, may protrude from the spine and push painfully against a nerve ending. In the past the treatment for this condition involved a major operation followed by a lengthy stay in a hospital. But now the treatment can be carried out under a local anesthetic. Probing with a needle 1 millimeter in diameter, the surgeon locates the damaged cartilage. Then the surgeon begins to slip a series of larger tubes over the needle to open a gap 3 millimeters to 7.5 millimeters across. Miniature retractors are pushed down the final tube to pull the nerve endings out of the way, and tiny burs are used to grind away any bone that may be trapping the nerve. Next a very small cutting tool is inserted into the cartilage to slice into it. Finally, a minute screw-shaped device is inserted into the spinal column to drain off fluid and relieve pressure. This causes the bones on either side of the disk to come together and fuse, leaving the patient a little shorter but no longer in pain.

an arm or a leg is relatively easy, but reconnecting numerous tiny severed blood vessels and nerves to restore full use of the limb calls for incredibly delicate techniques. These techniques are known as **microsurgery** because they must be carried out while the surgeon looks at the work area through a special surgical microscope that magnifies about 30 times.

At least eight stitches are needed to ensure a blood-tight connection between two sections of a severed blood vessel. The nylon thread used is narrower than a human hair and is attached to a fine needle 3 millimeters long made of the metal titanium. Although titanium costs much more than

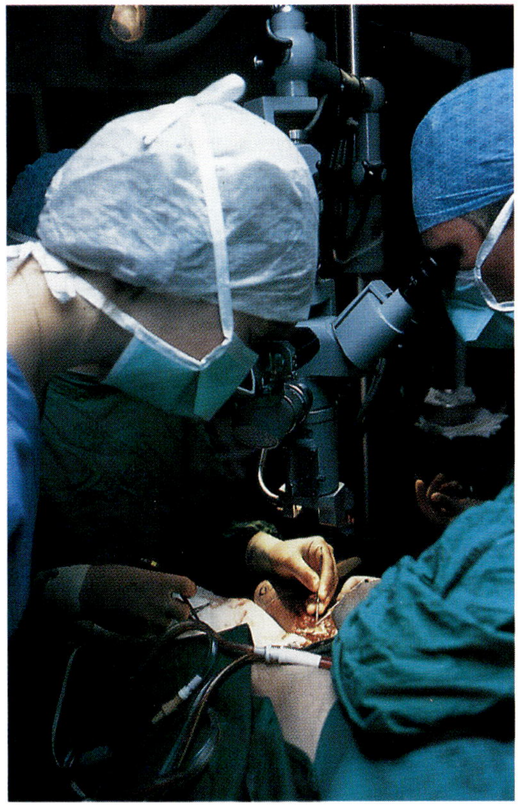

Two surgeons use an operating microscope and fine instruments to reconnect a patient's severed blood vessels.

steel, it is the only material that can be worked to a fine enough point.

Robo-Surgeon

The idea of a robot carrying out a delicate operation may sound terrifying, but the time is fast approaching when robots will take their place in the operating room alongside human surgeons. In fact, a robot has already successfully performed

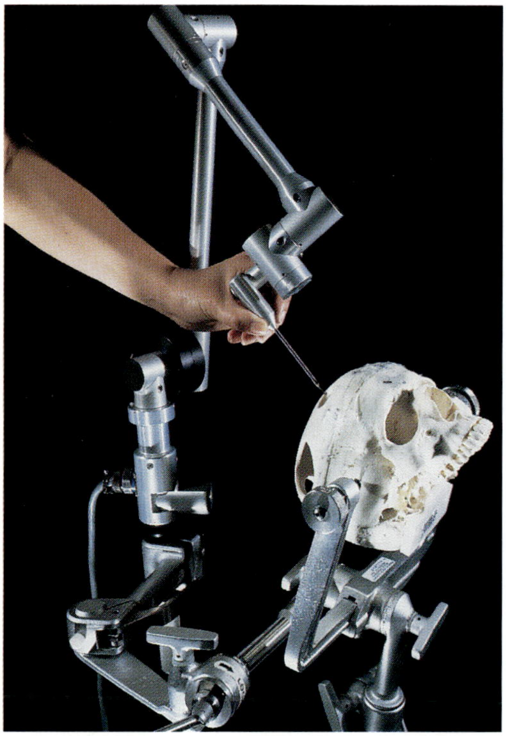

This hand-held robot arm with a probe is used to accurately locate brain tumors. CAT scan data of a patient's brain is fed into the robot's computer to create a three-dimensional image of the brain and tumor on a TV monitor. When the tip of the probe is moved on the patient's brain, the exact position of the tumor can be found while visualizing it on the screen.

surgery on an animal. In 1990 a ten-year-old sheepdog called Snook had its hip replaced at the University of California. A single-armed robot, programmed with the exact shape and size of the bone, used a rotary cutter to carve a cavity in the dog's thigh bone and then fitted the **implant.**

At first, robots that take part in operations on people will be used mainly for tasks that are simple but tedious for humans to perform. For instance, during keyhole surgery a miniature camera often has to be held for long periods by a junior doctor while the surgeon carries out the procedure. In

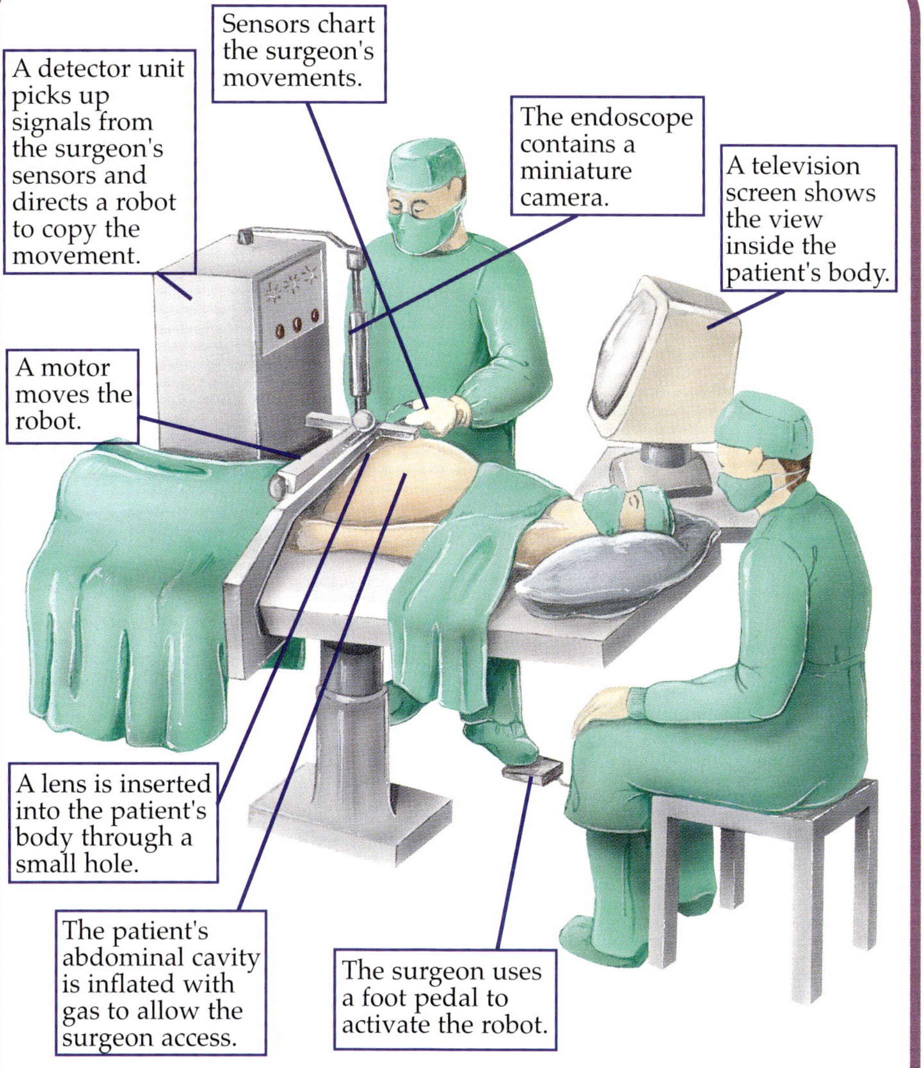

More and more operations in the future will be carried out by robots under the guidance of surgeons.

the future, robots will be used in such circumstances to handle the camera, freeing human assistants for more complex jobs.

Robots will also play an increasingly important role in operations that demand a high level of accuracy. In a typical future setup, the surgeon may not operate directly on the patient. Instead, sensory devices will track the movements of the surgeon and send signals to a detector unit. This unit, in turn, will control a motor attached to a robot holding a scalpel or other surgical tool so that the robot copies the surgeon's movements exactly. The equipment could also be arranged so that fairly large movements by the surgeon's hands are turned into smaller, more delicate actions by the robot.

Entering Inner Space

Even more amazing developments early in the next century could result in surgeons being outfitted more like astronauts than doctors. Work is going on to create a space-age helmet for surgeons that will display the interior of the patient's body. Wearing the helmet, the surgeon will have the impression of being inside the patient's heart or stomach or wherever else the operation site may be.

Special gloves equipped with electronic sensing gear will detect all movements of the surgeon's hands and transmit the movements to a miniature robot carrying tiny instruments inside the patient. With such equipment it would not even be necessary for the surgeon to be present in the operating room.

He or she could perform an operation remotely over a telephone line. This would allow a surgeon to operate on patients in different hospitals—even in different countries—from just one central location.

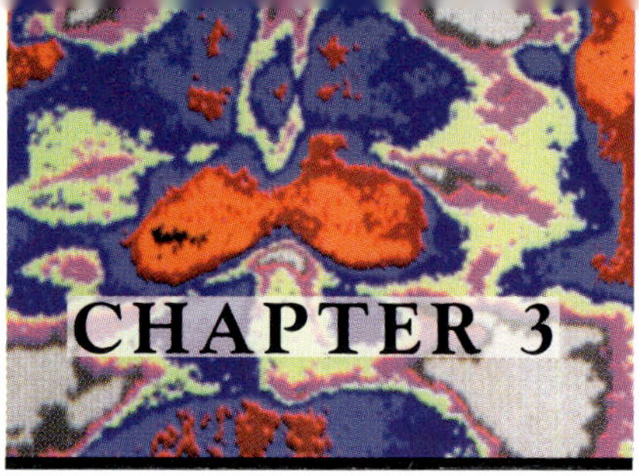

CHAPTER 3

Lifesaving Machines

Many people die needlessly each year simply because they don't receive medical treatment early enough. Further developments in such scanning methods as PET and MRI will mean that doctors will be able to detect the onset of life-threatening diseases at an earlier stage. Even the smallest of tumors will be found during routine scans and then, if necessary, will be treated by minimum-intervention methods before the tumors have a chance to threaten a patient's life.

More lives will also be saved in the future as a result of improvements in the speed and effectiveness of treatment given to accident and emergency victims. How soon a medical team can get to a critically ill patient and what resources are immediately at hand can make the difference between life and death for such patients.

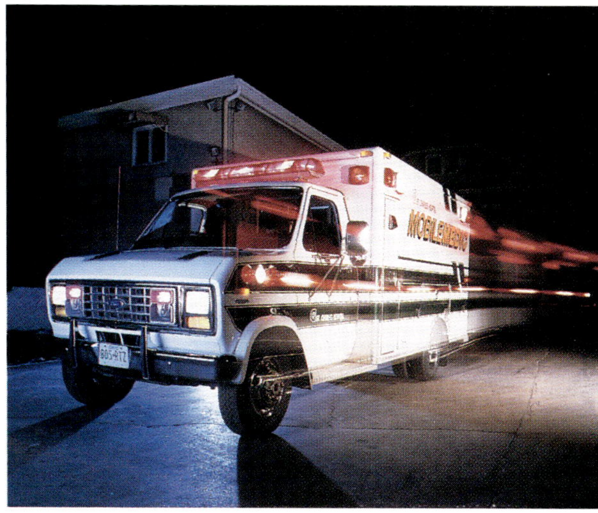

A modern ambulance, equipped with advanced lifesaving equipment, races to the scene of an accident.

Heart Restart

No medical emergency is more urgent than a sudden heart attack, or cardiac arrest. All at once and without warning, a person's heart stops beating properly and the flow of blood to the brain is cut off.

Even the short delay in getting a heart attack victim to a hospital may be too long. For this reason, ambulance crews are trained in two basic methods of revival. In the first, known as CPR (cardiopulmonary resuscitation), a medical technician breathes into the patient's mouth and presses on the chest repeatedly to keep the blood flowing and force oxygen as quickly as possible to the brain, heart, and other vital systems.

The emergency crew may also use a **defibrillator**. This device consists of two metal plates that can deliver a brief but powerful electric shock through the patient's heart. The sudden shock interrupts the random twitching of the heart muscles and stimulates the heart to resume its normal beating.

The difficulty is that too much time may pass before an expert is on hand to work an ordinary defibrillator. However, newly developed automatic defibrillators are helping to overcome this problem. The rescuer simply attaches sticky electrodes to the victim's chest and the automatic defibrillator does the rest. Programmed to measure the condition of the heart, it determines whether to give a shock. If a shock is needed, it determines where this shock should be directed and how strong it should be. A synthesized voice or visual display guides the rescuer in setting up the device.

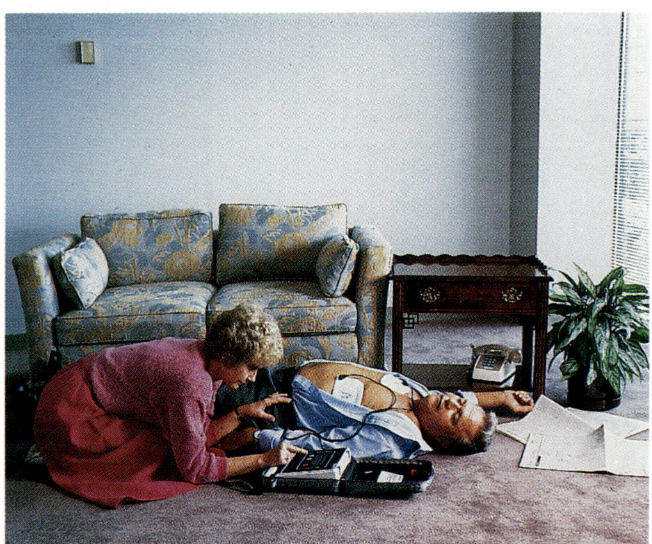

A heart attack victim being treated at home by a rescuer using an automatic defibrillator

Another recent development is the surgically implanted defibrillator. This is placed just under the skin of the patient's abdomen, where it continually monitors the heart's beating with a microcomputer. If the beats become weak and irregular, the device sends out a series of electrical pulses through fine wires leading to the heart. The pulses continue for 15 to 20 seconds. Since the pulses do not have to pass through the chest wall, they need only about one-fifteenth as much energy to control heartbeat as a normal defibrillator provides. The power source for the implant is a lithium battery that lasts about three years and can be replaced at regular intervals during a minor operation.

Monitors and Alarms

Doctors fighting to save the life of a critically ill or injured person rely on an array of instruments to continuously monitor the patient's breathing and heart condition. One of the most important tools at their disposal is the electrocardiograph (EKG).

The EKG works by sensing the weak electrical currents produced by muscles in the heart. These are transmitted to the machine through wires from a number of electrodes, which are smeared with conducting paste and fixed to the arms, legs, and chest. The EKG then amplifies the currents about 3,000 times and traces the patterns of heart waves on a screen or strip of paper.

A patient who is recovering from a heart attack or from cardiac surgery is connected to an EKG in the recovery room.

If the device senses that the heart is behaving abnormally, it instantly sounds an alarm at the nearest nurses' station.

One of the latest monitoring devices is the niroscope. This can show within two to three seconds whether the brain is receiving enough oxygen. Such a warning may be crucial, for example, while the patient is under an anesthetic. If deprived of oxygen for just three to four minutes, the brain would be permanently damaged.

The niroscope works by shining **infrared light** of different frequencies through the skull into the brain and measuring how much of that light is reflected back out. The operation of the niroscope is based on the fact that brain tissue absorbs different amounts of infrared light, depending on the amount of oxygen available to the brain cells.

Another valuable new tool is the echocardiograph. This instrument records the echoes of ultrasound waves from various parts of the heart. The instrument can show blood clots, faulty valves, and other abnormalities of the heart that might otherwise escape detection. One recent development of this technique involves the use of tiny sound transmitters that provide an even clearer image of the beating heart. The transmitters are located at the tip of an endoscope that is passed down the patient's throat. By altering the angle and position of the tip of the endoscope, the doctor can accurately direct ultrasound waves at a particular section of the heart and so obtain an image of that section while the heart is beating.

Machines That Changed Medicine

Stopping the heart long enough for surgery to be performed on it would once have been unthinkable. But this procedure is now routinely carried out, thanks to the development of the heart-lung machine. Blood from the patient is pumped into the machine. There the blood is supplied with oxygen—a task normally done by the lungs—and then passed back into the patient.

Another great medical breakthrough has been the construction of a machine to take over the role of the kidneys. These organs filter blood to remove impurities that, if allowed to accumulate, can seriously damage the body. Patients whose kidneys no longer work properly are connected to a kidney dialysis machine several times a week. The machine filters the blood artificially and returns the purified blood to the body. At first, dialysis machines were large, expensive, and in short supply, so difficult decisions had to be made concerning who would receive treatment and who would not. But advances in the technology of these devices have produced much smaller and less expensive machines that can be installed at home, which makes more machines available to more people.

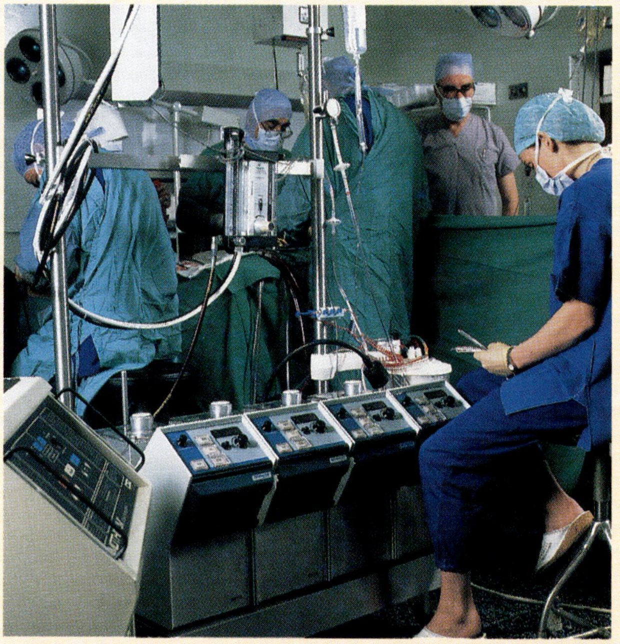

Surgeons perform surgery on a patient's heart while another doctor watches the heart-lung machine used to maintain the patient's circulation and vital functions during the operation.

Blasting Tumors

In the battle against cancer, doctors now have a variety of different weapons from which to choose. They can operate to cut away a tumor or burn it with a high-energy laser, treat the patient with a combination of cancer-destroying chemicals, or expose the diseased area to radiation.

Bathing a tumor in radiation from a radioactive source, however, has the side effect of damaging healthy tissue around

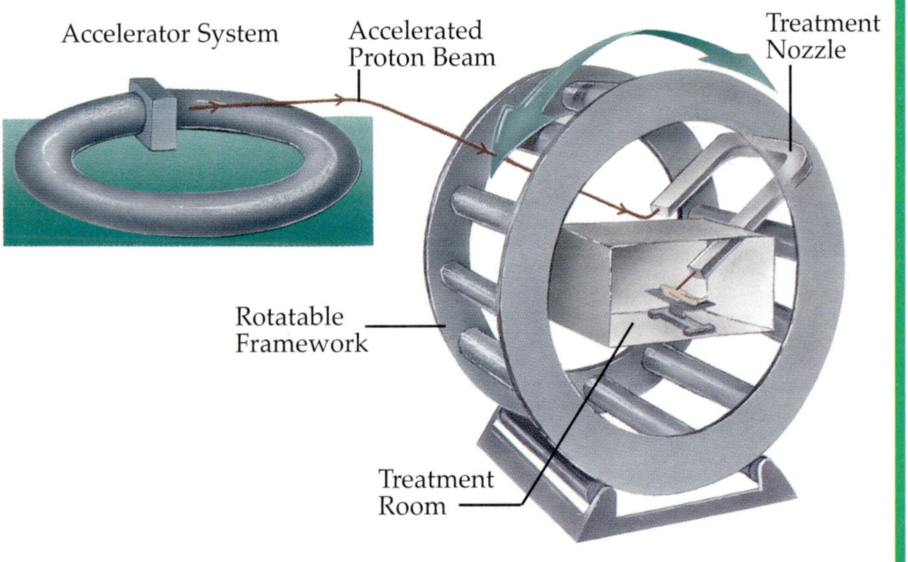

Proton accelerators show much promise in treating cancer. Powerful magnets create a magnetic field that accelerates protons to high speed. The protons can then be focused into a beam. The patient is placed inside a vast rotating wheel. The focused beam of protons breaks up the tumor, which is then excreted by the body. Healthy tissue near the tumor is not damaged.

the tumor. For this reason, much interest is being shown in a new form of cancer treatment involving **proton** beams.

Protons are positively-charged particles found inside the central part, or **nucleus**, of **atoms**. Being electrically charged, protons can be accelerated to high speed by a ring of powerful magnets inside a vast doughnut-shaped proton accelerator. Protons emerging from the accelerator can then be focused into a tight beam and fired with great accuracy down a nozzle at the diseased part of the patient's body.

The patient lies inside a giant rotating wheel that can direct the depth of the proton beam coming from the accelerator to within an accuracy of a few millimeters. Such fine targeting means that the maximum dose of radiation can be delivered to the tumor. As a result, the tumor is broken up and is then excreted by the body. Tissue lying in front of or behind the tumor, however, is left undamaged since it is not subjected to such an intense bombardment of protons.

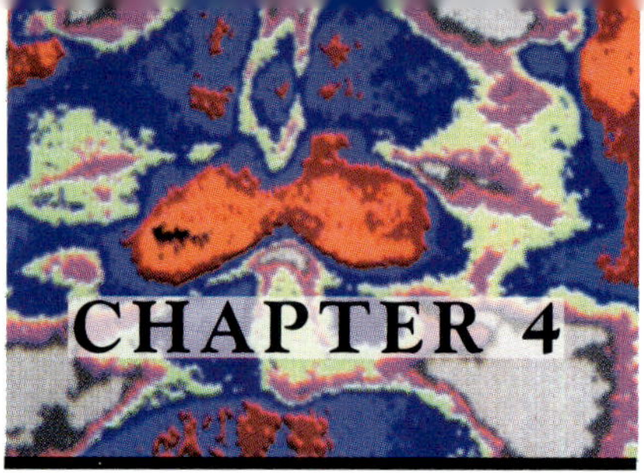

CHAPTER 4

New Parts for Old

When a part of the human body stops working through accident or disease, there is a good chance that modern surgery can replace it with either a natural or artificial substitute. The first transplant of an organ from one person to another took place on June 17, 1950, at a hospital in Chicago. A kidney from a woman who had just died was given to a 49-year-old woman named Ruth Tucker. Ten years later, in Cape Town, South Africa, Dr. Christiaan Barnard carried out the world's first heart transplant.

Since then, doctors have learned how to successfully transplant other organs, such as the liver, lungs, and pancreas. Meanwhile, researchers have developed a wide range of implants and prostheses—artificial body parts—to replace everything from hip joints to hands and feet.

Race Against Time

The biggest problem facing surgeons in transplanting an organ from one person (the donor) to another (the recipient) is tissue rejection. A transplant is rejected when the recipient's **immune system** attacks the cells of the transplant as it would any foreign invader, such as a virus or other disease-causing germ. Components of the blood known as white blood cells surround the cells of the foreign tissues and destroy them. If the body's defense system successfully attacks, or rejects, the cells of a transplanted organ, the organ dies.

To reduce the chance that this will happen, organs from potential donors are tested to see if their chemical properties are similar to those of the recipient. This step, known as tissue matching, helps to ensure that the recipient's defense system does not reject the transplanted organ.

Information about patients waiting for organ transplants, including their tissue types, is stored in a computer data bank. Then, when a donor becomes available—often following a fatal accident—the tissue type of the donor is determined and quickly matched against those of a number of possible recipients. If a match is found, the donor's organ is transported to the recipient's hospital. Donated organs must be healthy and preferably young, and they must be delivered to the transplant surgeon as rapidly as possible. After being removed from the donor, the organ is quickly pumped full of fluid to prevent blood clots from forming. Then it is packed in ice and put in a cold storage container at 40°F (5°C).

Speed is essential in transporting the organ to the hospital where the transplant will be carried out. An ice-packed heart becomes useless after 3 to 5 hours, a liver after 10 hours, and a kidney after 24 to 48 hours. Researchers are working to develop special chemicals and new forms of storage that will extend the life of donated organs to many days or even weeks.

Mending Broken Hearts

Far more people need new organs than there are donors available. For this reason, one of the long-range goals of medical technology is to develop complete artificial substitutes for various organs, especially the heart.

During the 1980s, there were 90 people around the world who were fitted with a type of artificial heart called the Jarvik-7, which worked by means of compressed air. One American man, who received his new heart in 1986, survived for 20 months. But the suffering he went through after his operation received a lot of publicity. Doctors and other people debated about whether any more Jarvik hearts should be implanted in patients until more advanced technology became available. Then, at the end of 1989, artificial heart surgery was banned in the United States.

Since that time, researchers have concentrated mainly on improving devices that will assist a damaged heart or take the place of a small section of the heart or blood vessel that is no longer able to do its job properly. For example, diseased arteries—large blood vessels that carry blood away from the heart—can be replaced by new ones made of polyurethane. Damaged heart valves that regulate the flow of blood into and out of the heart and between the heart's chambers can be replaced by valves made of plastic or metal alloy. Meanwhile, scientists continue research to reach the long-range goal of developing total artificial substitutes for such organs as the heart. The artificial organs, however, must be perfected so that they are acceptable to surgeons, patients, and society.

Setting the Pace

The most common implant used to help the heart is the artificial pacemaker. Normally the heart has its own pacemaker, which produces an electrical impulse along special conducting fibers. When this wave of electrical stimulation spreads across the heart tissue, it causes the muscles of the heart to contract in sequence, pumping blood around the body.

Some diseases interfere with the functions of the heart's natural pacemaker. In such a case, the heart is unable to contract properly. One treatment of this condition involves the implanting of an artificial pacemaker. The artificial pacemaker takes over the job of the defective natural one and, thus, restores normal heart function. The artificial pacemaker is a small electrical unit that is installed under the skin of a patient's chest. Wires from the pacemaker are connected to the

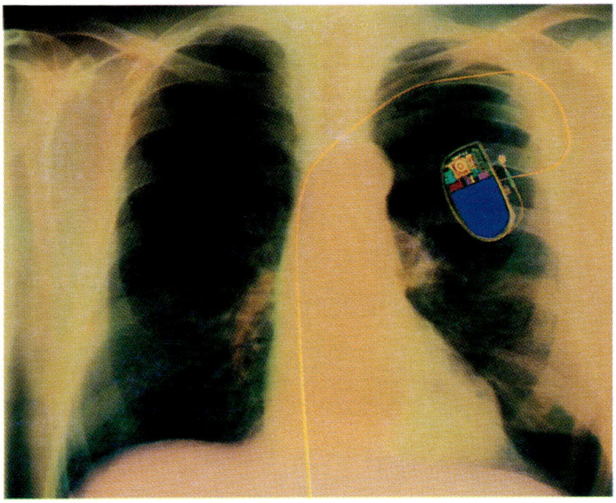

A colored X-ray of a patient's chest, showing a fitted pacemaker. This electronic battery-run device is seen above the rib cage, with a yellow lead that connects it to the heart.

heart itself. The wires carry electrical impulses that stimulate the heart so that it beats normally.

Great progress has been made since the first artificial pacemaker was constructed in 1958. The batteries used to power the earliest models had to be replaced every two years or so. In contrast, in 1988 a 47-year-old man was fitted with a nuclear pacemaker containing a tiny pellet of the radioactive material plutonium. The pellet held enough energy to run the pacemaker for at least 20 years. **Microprocessors** of ever-increasing power are also being attached to pacemakers so that the stimulating signals sent to the heart can be finely adjusted from one beat to the next, depending on the heart's condition. In the future, artificial pacemakers will be able to perform almost as well as their healthy, natural counterparts, while the fuel sources that supply them will last a lifetime.

Artificial Joints

Joints may wear out or become diseased as people grow older, and limbs may become paralyzed through illness or accident. In such cases, modern surgery can often come to the rescue with an impressive array of high-technology replacement parts.

One of the most common operations today is the total replacement of a hip joint. Every year over 100,000 people in the United States and a similar number in Europe are given new hip joints made of steel and a special hard-wearing plastic. The operation involves gouging out the socket of the joint and replacing it with a plastic cup. At the same time, the head of the femur—the long bone in the upper leg whose ball fits

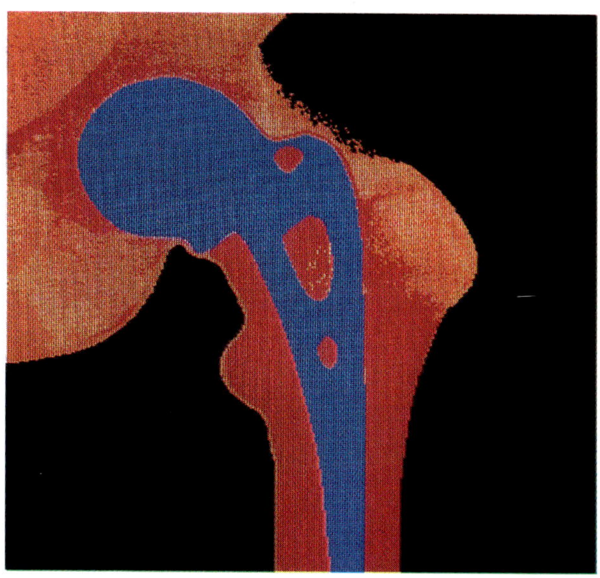

A false-color X-ray of a patient's pelvis, showing an artificial hip joint

into the hip socket—is removed and replaced by a metal head. Extending from this metal head is a long stem, which is cemented into a hole drilled into the rest of the femur.

Developing a successful artificial joint such as a hip replacement is much more difficult than it seems. A natural joint can perform well for 70 to 80 years and has its own lubrication system that makes the areas of contact slipperier than ice on ice. To provide an adequate substitute, surgeons and engineers must try out all sorts of designs and combinations of materials until they find an arrangement that will do the job. In the future their efforts will be helped by increasingly powerful computers that can accurately model the forces joints are subjected to and also by the creation of new materials that will extend the lifetime of replacement parts.

Walking with the Computer's Help

Some people lose the use of their legs because of spinal injuries. However, many of these people can now be helped to stand and walk again by using a new computer-aided technique. Electrodes are fastened to a patient's legs, and braces are strapped on to support each knee joint. Wires run from the electrodes to a computer-controlled device that can deliver short electric pulses. Every time a pulse is sent out along a wire, it stimulates the movement of one particular muscle in one of the patient's legs. The computer is programmed with the sequence in which pulses must be transmitted to cause first one leg to take a step and then the other. Progress in learning to walk using this system is often difficult and slow, but it offers real hope to patients who might otherwise be confined to a wheelchair for the rest of their lives.

Restoring Movement

Victims of accidents who suffer damage to their limbs as well as people paralyzed for various reasons can now benefit from some extraordinary developments in the design of artificial arms, legs, hands, and feet. For example, people who have undergone amputation of an arm above the elbow can be given an artificial arm that works under electronic control. Tiny electrodes are attached to muscles in the upper arm or shoulder. These electrodes conduct signals from the muscles to the artificial arm so that it can be moved up and down. In the same way, signals can be conveyed from the muscles to vary the firmness

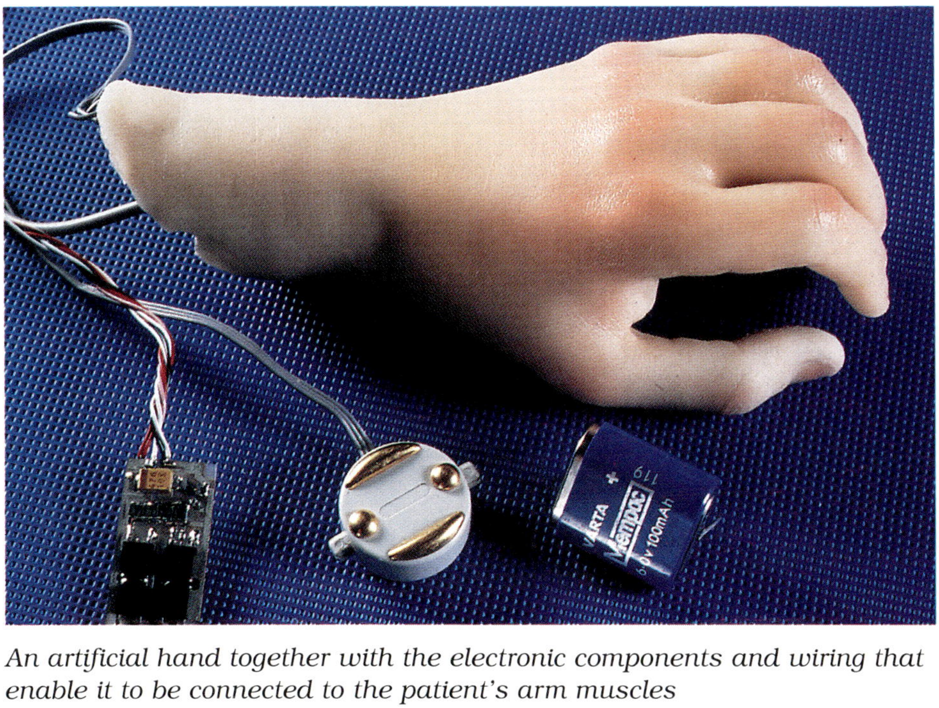

An artificial hand together with the electronic components and wiring that enable it to be connected to the patient's arm muscles

of grip of an artificial hand so that it can be used, for example, to pick up an egg or a delicate glass without crushing it.

Equipped with the latest kinds of artificial limbs, people are able to walk, run, lift, and carry just as if they had natural arms and legs. They can even be given a sense of feeling and touch in their new limbs.

The most advanced kind of artificial leg uses devices called transducers, which are placed in the sole of the artificial foot. These transducers send electrical signals to electrodes attached to the skin of the wearer's stump. As many as eight electrodes, each connected to a separate transducer, are attached to a special stump socket that fits precisely against the person's remaining thighbone and muscles. The healthy muscles and nerves in the stump pick up the transducers' signals and transmit them to the brain as if they were coming from a natural foot. The brain interprets the messages as varying degrees of pressure on different parts of the sole. This gives the wearer of such an artificial leg a limited sense of feeling, which in turn allows the person better control over leg and foot movements.

Future developments in the field of artificial limbs will allow users more sensitive feelings in their artificial hands and feet. They will be able to detect changes in texture and temperature and may eventually find it hard to tell the difference between the living parts of their bodies and those that are artificial.

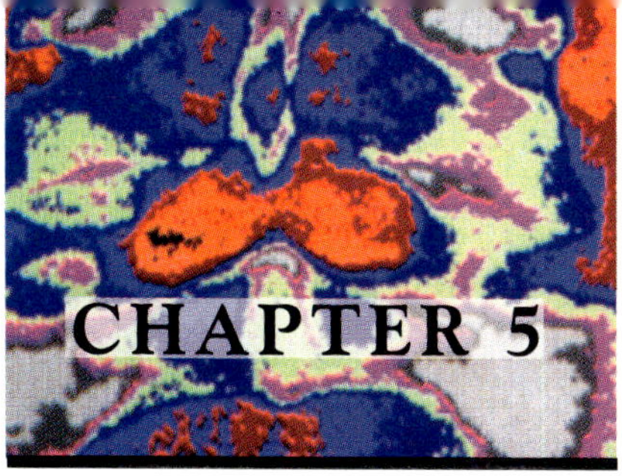

CHAPTER 5

Restoring Sight and Hearing

Until recently, very little could be done to help people who were blind or profoundly deaf. But now medical science has developed a number of ways to restore partial hearing or sight to those who have lost or have never been able to use these senses.

One of the simplest of the new techniques is to replace a defective lens in the eye with a plastic substitute. For a variety of reasons, the natural lens in a person's eye may become cloudy. This cloudiness, known as a **cataract**, stops light from entering the eye and in severe cases results in almost total blindness. To correct the problem, with the aid of a microscope a surgeon opens up the clear part of the front of the eye—the **cornea**. The surgeon then removes the patient's diseased lens, which lies behind the cornea. Next, an artificial lens is put in the place of the natural one.

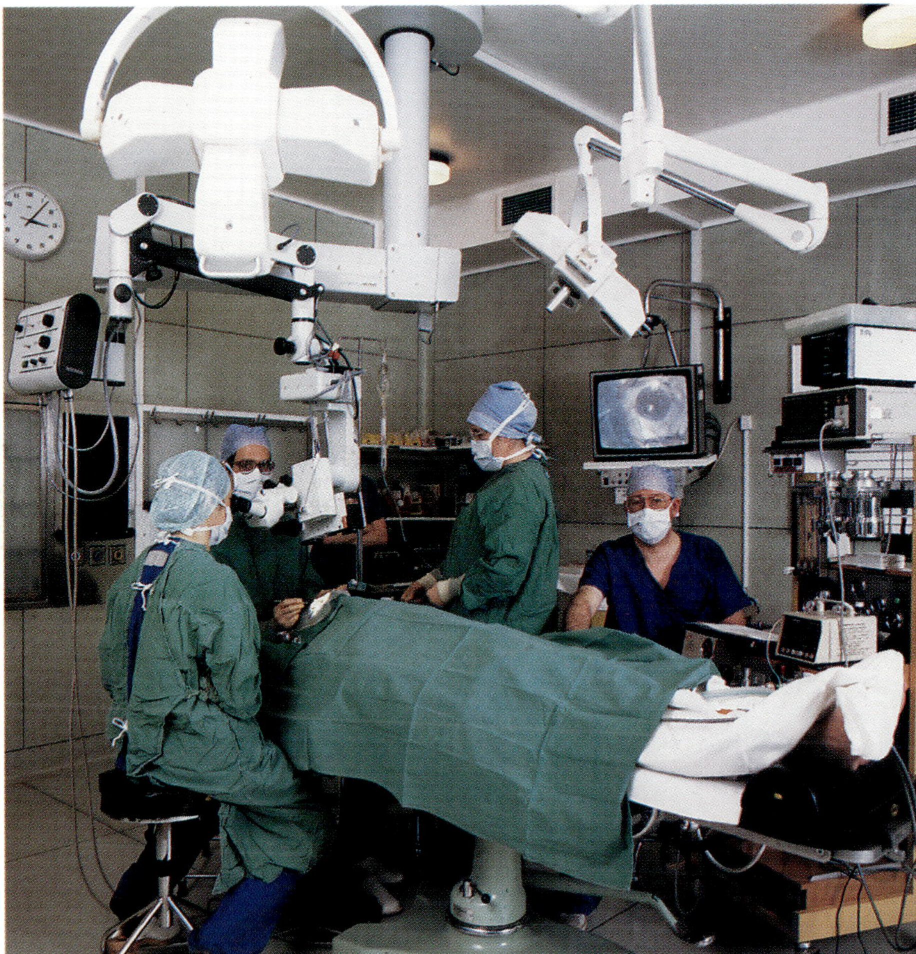

An eye operation being carried out with microsurgical techniques. A close-up of the patient's eye, as seen through the surgeon's microscope, appears on the monitor.

Sight Repairs

A number of other operations are now routinely carried out to repair damage to the eyes and restore normal vision. At the back of the eye is a light-sensitive layer called the **retina**. The cells of the retina transmit vision signals to cells behind the retina. If the retina becomes torn or detached through an accident or disease, a person may become partly or completely blind. However, by using a narrow laser beam, a surgeon can effectively weld the damaged areas back into place.

Specialized lasers play an important part in the treatment of a serious eye condition known as **glaucoma**. In glaucoma, the pressure of the liquid inside the eyeball increases until it threatens to destroy a person's sight. By shining a laser through the cornea and burning a tiny hole in it, a surgeon can relieve the buildup of pressure without having to make a cut into the eye.

Damage to the cornea—the tough, clear outer covering of the center of the eye—can sometimes be repaired by a corneal transplant. This involves replacing the damaged section with a piece of healthy cornea taken from the eye of a donor. The operation calls for the finest stitches of any that are used in surgery, with suture thread no thicker than a human hair and needles less than a quarter of an inch long.

In 1995, surgeons in the United States began testing a bionic eye, which contains a miniature black and white TV camera. Signals are carried from the camera by a wire under the skin to a particular area of the skull. This area lies over the part of the brain that processes visual signals. The wire is attached to 256 tiny electrodes, each fitted to a small cluster of brain cells. In this way, it is hoped, electronic impulses from the camera will create visual images in the brain.

Hear, Hear

People who have limited hearing can have sounds made louder by a hearing aid. But just because the sounds are louder doesn't necessarily mean they are clearer. The problem is that ordinary hearing aids amplify all the sounds they pick up by the same amount. They don't allow for the fact that deafness affects different people in different ways.

Very often, people who are deaf can hear some frequencies of sound better than others. The frequency of sound determines pitch. For example, a high-frequency note has a high pitch. A low-frequency note has a low pitch. Deafness usually affects sounds of higher pitch more than sounds of lower pitch, which makes understanding speech, in particular, very difficult. To help get around this problem, researchers have developed hearing aids that can amplify some sounds more than others.

Important work in this field is being carried out at, among other places, the University of New Mexico in Albuquerque. The work is based on 30 years of investigation by scientists in the former Yugoslavia. These researchers studied the relationship between the understanding of speech and the frequencies of speech sounds. They also studied how different languages produce different sound frequencies. Based on their findings, the Yugoslav researchers developed a hearing aid that amplified sounds only at certain frequencies. Scientists at the University of New Mexico took this idea further by introducing computer technology so that the hearing aid could be reprogrammed to meet the needs of different users or the characteristics of different languages. The scientists called their invention the digital master hearing aid, or DMHA.

The first version of the DMHA, built in 1992, was about the size of a personal stereo, weighed just over 2 pounds, and was connected to a headset by a wire. The hearing aid worked using a special **microchip** that acted as a **signal processor** to boost the level of incoming sounds at selected frequencies. In the future the DMHA and devices like it will be developed further so that they are smaller and lighter and are linked to the wearer's headset by radio signals instead of wires. A person requiring a hearing aid will visit a specialist and have his or her hearing tested across a wide range of frequencies. The information gathered from the test will be stored in a **memory chip**. Then the memory chip will be inserted into the hearing aid to customize it to the particular needs of the wearer. The memory chip will tell the signal-processing chip how much to boost the volume at each frequency to give the user a sense of hearing that is as near to normal as possible.

Journey of a Sound Wave

The fleshy outside part of the ear, called the pinna, collects sounds and helps us identify the direction from which they come. The sound waves then travel down the auditory canal to the eardrum, a membrane that forms a barrier between the outer and the middle ear. When sound waves strike it, the eardrum vibrates, like the skin of a drum. Its vibrations are transmitted across the air-filled middle ear by the three smallest bones in the ear—the hammer, anvil, and stirrup. The stirrup is connected to a thin membrane, known as the oval window, which is set into the snail-shaped **cochlea** of the inner ear. Vibrations of the oval window are detected by over 20,000 tiny hairs inside the cochlea. As these hairs vibrate, they stimulate nerve cells at their base. Signals from these nerve cells go up the auditory nerve to the brain, allowing us to hear. Joined to the cochlea are three semicircular canals, filled with fluid and set at right angles to one another, which help control our balance.

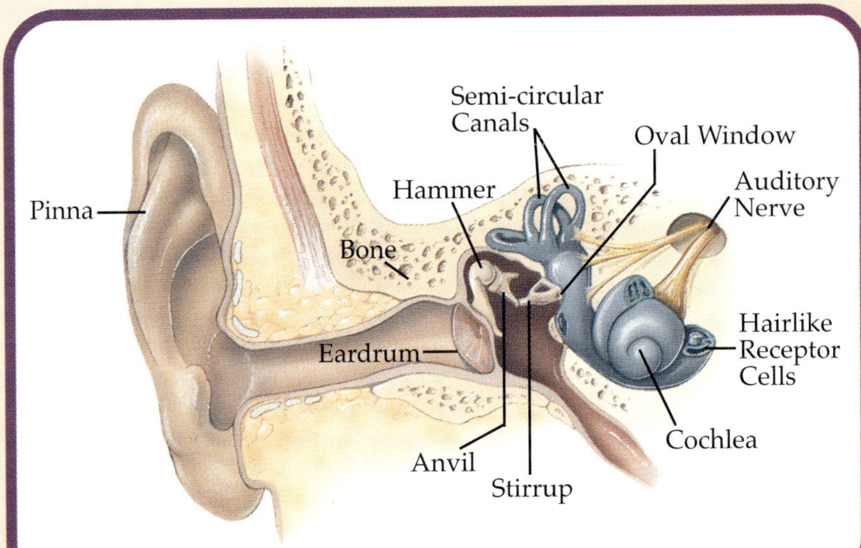

Inside the human ear

Artificial Ears

The outer part of the ear is the simplest. When something goes wrong with the complicated parts that are hidden from view—the middle ear and the inner ear—then corrective action becomes difficult. In fact, until a few years ago, to replace parts of the middle or inner ear would have been beyond the surgeon's power. Now, however, thousands of people every year are having their hearing at least partially restored, thanks to artificial implants.

As a result of a recent development in Japan, patients suffering from inflammation of the eardrum or middle ear can be given an artificial middle ear. Normally, sound passes down the channel of the outer ear to the eardrum. The eardrum vibrates, and the sound vibration is transmitted by three tiny bones in the middle ear to the cochlea.

The artificial middle ear developed in Japan bypasses the eardrum and the first two bones of the middle ear. Part of the device hooks behind the outside of the ear and converts sounds into magnetic signals that are picked up by a second component implanted within the skull. This second component transmits the signals along a wire to a vibrator placed in the middle-ear cavity. The vibrator then moves the third bone, known as the stirrup, which passes on this movement to the cochlea.

Cochlear Implants

Another new type of implant, called a cochlear implant,

bypasses the eardrum and middle ear altogether and stimulates the cochlea directly. It can help give people who are totally deaf some form of hearing, provided they have intact nerve fibers connecting the cochlea to the brain.

The cochlear implant consists of a tiny disk-shaped radio receiver with a long tail containing very fine wires. Dotted along the tail are a number of electrodes—little pieces of metal out of which an electric current can pass. A surgeon places the receiver beneath the skin, just behind the ear, and pushes the tail of the implant around the snail-like curl of the cochlea.

Outside the ear is a microphone that picks up sound. The

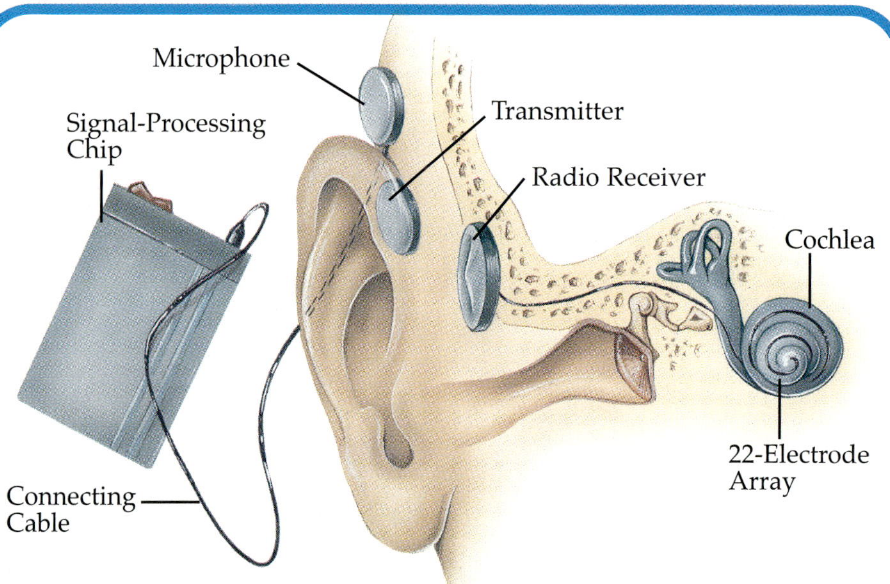

The cochlear implant—a device that has already restored partial hearing to thousands of people around the world

signal is passed to a signal-processing chip that converts the sound into electrical impulses. These impulses are then sent to a tiny transmitter that sits behind the ear directly over the receiver. When the receiver picks up the processed sound signals, it passes them down to the electrode inside the cochlea.

The earliest type of cochlear implant had only one electrode on the tail and was known as a single-channel implant. It stimulated the nerve fibers and sent just one electrical signal to the brain. The signal matched the sound waves picked up by the microphone, but it was left to the brain to try to sort out the frequency patterns, a job normally done by the cochlea.

More recent implants have a string of 22 or more electrodes along the tail, resting at different places in the cochlea. These multichannel devices depend on more sophisticated signal-processing chips that analyze the frequency pattern of sounds picked up by the microphone. Signals representing different sound frequencies are then sent to different parts of the cochlea, so the implant works in a manner closer to that of the natural ear.

Developments to Come

As miniature computers become ever more powerful, it will be possible to make replacement parts for ears and eyes that give a better and better quality of hearing and vision. Cochlear implants, for example, may eventually be able to analyze sounds in as much detail as a healthy human cochlea and so restore a person's hearing to normal. Similar advances in technology that allow visual scenes to be broken down into fine parts and turned into signals that can be fed along the optic nerve directly to the brain will allow blind people to see clearly.

Over the next few decades, it will become increasingly common for people to have defective or worn-out natural body parts replaced by artificial ones. This will allow accident victims, disabled people, and elderly people to live fuller, healthier, and longer lives.

But advances in surgery and medical care will also create a number of problems. The proportion of people of advanced age will steadily rise, which will place a strain on facilities that care for the elderly. The ability of people to pay for expensive implants may determine who is treated and who is not. And, finally, there is the ethical question of how much of a human being we are willing to replace by machinery. When it becomes possible, as it almost certainly will, to replace eyes, ears, and even parts of the brain by electronic devices, will we want to place limits on what the surgeon should and should not do? If such limits are not imposed, will the time eventually come when, after repeated surgery, some people are more artificial than natural? And should that matter? These are questions that will need to be given serious consideration as we move into the next century.

Glossary

Alzheimer's disease—A progressive deterioration of the brain, most common in elderly people, that results in a loss of memory and a general breakdown in mental and physical health.

atom—A basic particle of matter. All substances are made of atoms, which are often combined to make larger units called molecules. Inside each atom are smaller particles known as protons, neutrons, and electrons.

blood transfusion—The replacement of blood lost by a patient by other blood of the same type or a compatible type.

CAT—The technique of computerized axial tomography, which directs a series of X-ray beams through the body to produce detailed cross sections.

cataract—A cloudiness of the lens of the eye, which can lead to blindness. It is common in old age and may also result from an illness such as diabetes.

cochlea—The spiral-shaped structure in the inner ear in which sound vibrations of different frequencies are turned into nerve impulses before being sent to the brain.

cornea—The transparent, protective outer covering of the center of the eye.

defibrillator—A device that can be used to restart the heart by producing a strong electric shock across a patient's chest.

digital images—Pictures built up from many separate points, each point representing an item of data that has been collected by an instrument and stored as a number inside a computer.

Doppler scanning—A scanning technique that uses ultrasound to measure the speed of moving objects, for example, the blood inside the body.

electrode—A conducting part, usually made of metal, by which an electric current leaves or enters a device.

endoscope—A long, flexible device equipped with a light, a lens, and various instruments that can be used to look inside the body and carry out certain types of surgery.

fetus—An unborn child from the end of the eighth week of pregnancy to the moment of birth. Before the eighth week the unborn child is known as an embryo.

forceps—Pincers used by surgeons for a variety of purposes, such as holding back tissues or pinching off severed blood vessels to prevent bleeding.

frequency—When applied to waves such as sound waves, light waves, or radio waves, it is the number of vibrations, or waves, that pass a point in one second.

glaucoma—A disease in which the pressure of the liquid inside the eyeball increases above normal. Unless treated in time, the disease causes irreparable damage to a person's sight.

hydrogen atom—The smallest particle of hydrogen. Hydrogen atoms are very common in many substances and tissues in the human body.

immune system—The body's chemical defense system, which is used to identify and destroy foreign invaders, such as viruses.

implant—An artificial part or device that is placed inside the human body to take the place of a natural part that has been damaged by accident or disease.

infrared light—Light similar to ordinary light but invisible and consisting of waves of lower frequency. We experience infrared light as heat waves.

keyhole surgery—Surgery that is carried out through small cuts and openings about the size of a thumbnail.

magnetic field—The region around a magnet where the effects of the magnet are exerted.

memory chip—A microchip that is used to store information for use by a computer.

microchip—A complex circuit made from microscopic components, laid down on a single crystal of a substance called silicon, that can store or process information.

microprocessor—A microchip that works as the processing section of a computer.

microsurgery—Surgery so delicate that it requires the use of a surgical microscope and miniature instruments.

minimum-intervention—A term used to describe surgery that attempts to treat the patient while causing as little damage to the body as possible.

MRI—The technique of magnetic resonance imaging. A patient in an MRI scanner is surrounded by a strong magnet and exposed to high-frequency radio waves. This causes the nuclei of hydrogen atoms to give off radio waves at a certain frequency that the scanner is set up to detect.

nucleus—The central part of an atom, which contains most of its mass. The nucleus consists of protons and (except for atoms of ordinary hydrogen) neutrons.

optical fiber—A fine, bendable strand of specially made glass or plastic in which light can easily travel.

organ—A part of the body, built up from various types of tissue, that performs a unique, important task. Examples of organs include the heart, the brain, the lungs, the stomach, and the kidneys.

percutaneous surgery—A new type of surgical procedure that involves operating through needle-sized holes.

PET—The technique of positron emission tomography. This involves injecting a patient with a radioactive sugar solution and then using a PET scanner to measure how much of the sugar has been absorbed by different parts of the patient's brain.

proton—A very small positively charged particle found within the nuclei of atoms.

radioactive—Emitting penetrating rays and particles of several types due to the breakup of the nuclei of certain atoms.

retina—The layer at the back of the eye that senses the intensity and color of light.

retractor—A tool used in surgery to hold back parts, such as bones and muscles, that would otherwise get in the way of the operation.

scalpel—A very sharp, lightweight knife used in surgery.

signal processor—A device used to distinguish and separate the different parts that make up a sound or other kind of signal.

tissue—A group of similar cells that perform a specific and common function. For example, a section of muscle, a section of skin, and a part of an organ are tissues.

transplant—The replacement of a diseased or defective organ, or part of an organ, with a healthy organ taken from another person.

tumor—An abnormal growth in some part of the body.

ultrasound—Sound consisting of waves of very high frequency.

X-rays—High-frequency electromagnetic waves that can be used to take pictures of structures inside the body.

For Further Reading

Bender, Lionel, *Frontiers of Medicine* (Through the Microscope series). Watts, 1991.

Cassedy, James H. *Medicine in America: A Short History* (American Moments series). John Hopkins, 1991.

Curtis, Robert. *Great Lives: Medicine*. Macmillan, 1992.

Darling, David. *Computers of the Future: Intelligent Machines and Virtual Reality* (Beyond 2000 series). Dillon Press, 1996.

Fradin, Dennis B. *Medicine: Yesterday, Today, & Tomorrow* (Twentieth Century Science & Beyond series). Childrens, 1989.

Garell, Dale C. and Synder, Solomon H., eds. *Medical Technology* (Medical Issues series). Chelsea House, 1993.

Hawkes, Nigel. *Medicine & Health* (New Technology series). TFC Books.

Hooper, Tony. *Surgery* (Breakthrough series). Raintree Steck-Vaughn, 1993.

O'Neil, Karen E. *Health and Medicine Projects for Young Scientists* (Projects for Young Scientists series). Watts, 1993.

Power, Vicki. *Medicine & Health* (New Directions series). Watts, 1992.

Senior, Kathryn. *Medicine: Doctors, Demons & Drugs* (Timelines series). Watts, 1993.

Youngson, Robert M. Surgery Book: Seventy-five of the Most Common Operations Illustrated and Explained. St. Martin's Press, 1993.

Index